# Reflexology and her sister Yoga

## Evie Fleming

# ABOUT THE AUTHOR

Well I was born in a little log cabin in South Carolina. No... Just kidding. But I am a Carolina girl. My family was a nice middle-class family by society standards. I was born during the 60s. A few months before my birth, President Kennedy was assassinated. Then four years later, Martin Luther King. I can only imagine how it was for my parents and their daily struggles with the battles of civil rights, race riots and then the essential signing of the Civil Rights Act of 1964.

My little soul came into this world where there was a lot of unrest and a drive to get a man on the moon. We as humans were striving to expand beyond our universe. I wonder how I sought out peace and stillness in those moments. Was this the precursor, a driving force that led me to certifications in reflexology and yoga? My journey for balance, peace and stillness.

I can't remember my family having any exercise regime. No gym memberships. No workout benches in the house. My father played baseball and tennis. We were very active as kids but the most we played were outdoor activities in the front yard with cousins, enjoying recess time on the playground of school or the neighborhood park. I did not join any athletic teams during my early school years but I participated in gym activities. I finally decided that cheerleading was the way to go. You get a free ride to all school athletic events and you get to be front and center. I loved the team energy more than anything the emotional high when your team is winning!

As far as a spiritual or religious background I was baptized and confirmed in the Episcopal church of my grandmother. She came for us every Sunday without fail, sometimes knocking on the door until we answered and staying until we got dressed. She was determined. My siblings and I can laugh for hours about time spent in church pews trying not to get the attention of my grandmother. Boy, if she came down from the choir and grabbed you, well let's say you didn't talk the same when you returned. My parents, however, never pushed the issue of church. Later in life I would explore and come in contact with many denominations. I learned what it means to be: Baptist, Jehovah's Witness, Evangelical, Sufi, Unitarian, Mennonite, Jewish, Muslim, and a Buddhist. In retrospect, I can see I was seeking out one way that resonated with my soul. Ultimately all paths lead to the one... Or is that the matrix? I digress.

Our souls are always gathering information. Making moves to lead us to our purpose or mission in this lifetime. I am glad to have found something I love and that is good for my body and soul. I enjoy sharing new reflexology tips and helping friends when they say "hey do you know a yoga pose for this?" It feels right to me and it is why I always encourage my clients to always stay connected on the inner planes.

Always asking... How does it feel in the body?

# CHAPTER 1

# YOU SHOULD BE A YOGA TEACHER!

These were words spoken to me by one of my favorite Yoga Teachers Michele Ludtke. I want to take a moment and take you back to my journey to that time, but first let's have a brief intro to yoga (my understanding of it).

Yoga was developed over 5,000 years ago in India. It started as a practice with rituals and mantras. Individuals sought to rise to a higher level. This was done with discipline and a consistent practice of developing from the inside out. Yes the asanas/poses were present, but not the main focus. Later, people began to use the physical aspect more as a way to get the body to release unwanted stressors or unwanted energy. The belief was swinging, and this shift was moving toward a higher consciousness. This movement has birthed the Yoga we know here in the western world.

I, like most of us, believe that any good workout must leave you sweating or breathing hard. You have to feel the burn of the body to call it a true workout. So the first time I went to yoga it was as a way to work out. It was the new and happening thing. I am going to date myself with these next few statements but here we go: My initiation was the VHS tape. Yep, VHS! Some of you will say, *what*? Others will know how old I am. OK. stop giggling and let me finish my story. So I get my mat and my cute little leggings and pop the tape in and turn on the TV. I start to follow along, work to get in a quiet space.

Mom!! (A yell from outside my bedroom)

Well that didn't last long. Of course I am in my bedroom and I have two young kids, so the quiet doesn't last as they wander in one by one to see what I am up to. They began to show me they can bend and twist like pretzels. Needless to say it took me a few days to even get through that one-hour tape. Once finished, if someone asked about yoga, I could now say, "yes, I have done yoga." (LOL NOT)

I think I got a few more tapes and continued to do my own practice at home. It took a few years before I actually took a formal class at a gym. I, like many, joined the gym at the New Year, making my resolution to do better and live healthy. I liked yoga at the gym because it built a sense of being in it with others. You get to see people struggle like you do or get to feel proud when you can touch your toes and others cannot. So crazy how competitive we can be in any situation. Again, other things took a front seat and my days at the gym didn't last long, but my interest in yoga stayed with me.

Many years later my return to the fitness arena came through a partnership with Meeka. We decided to be workout buddies and accountability partners. I am not an early riser so we first started later, after work. Then she convinced me that by going early we could get it done and it would be a great start to the day. So we tried an early morning routine before heading into work at 8 AM. I eventually found my way to yoga again. I think it is a good idea to really explore different classes and teachers to allow time to see how your body responds. You don't know what you will like until you try it. Yoga is a body experience, beyond the mind.

With yoga there are several styles you could try: Vinyasa flow, ashtanga, hot yoga, restorative and Iyengar. There's an abundance of approaches. These are just a few. So get curious and explore.

This is exactly what I did. I have tried many different styles and attended classes with various teachers. Each has their own unique way of doing things, and I can tell you that you will gravitate toward the teacher that resonates with you. So exploring and seeking is definitely a part of the yoga experience. Teaching you to color a bit outside the lines and establishing your own individual foundation.

After being a student for a while and attending classes at my favorite fitness club, I was in the locker room unwinding from a great yoga session. My yoga teacher Michele came up and said to me how great I was doing and then landed those words: "you should be a Yoga Teacher." (I, of course, smiled and shrugged, thinking she was just flattering me. But I was sold on her class. Definitely a follower and will always recommend her.) She saw my disbelief and said, "Seriously, you should consider it. We are offering a training here soon. Please take a look and sign up." Wow! Of course my head was spinning. Flattering thought, but I am not a teacher. I'm constantly hearing the voice in my head and often from others about how I don't speak up, I don't use my voice. Now she is suggesting I use it to teach. OK, I'm going to need a minute.

After much back-and-forth conversation with myself, and a roller coaster ride of emotions, I signed up. I am not going to go into the details about which program I took because we all should decide for ourselves. But I will say it was an easy weekend course, and it allowed me to get my feet wet to understand the mechanics of teaching and level-one yoga. They laid out the class format and we got to practice. My first attempt to teach was a volunteer assignment for a women's shelter. In some ways this was Grace as I look back on it. I got a chance to come out of my shell and face my fear of teaching. How? Because I was giving of myself in service to someone else. These women were at a critical time in their lives and it was my assignment to give them a moment of release. So with that in mind I was all-in. I am forever grateful for my time there.

My journey with yoga had me take a few more weekend courses and eventually I began to teach at some area fitness clubs. Teaching in that environment can be intimidating. I remember how students would leave in the middle of class or talk to me after about other teachers' classes they liked and how I should check it out. (Hint! Hint!) But eventually I found my own way, my student numbers grew, and I began to have fun with my classes and made them my own. To have my students come up to me and say, "good class," was great validation.

However, I was near completion and I decided to shift gears and enroll in a year-long immersion of yoga under another teacher. I know it sounds crazy, why shift? I am a person who follows signs. I had been contemplating going forward to complete my certification. I was planning my next classes, locations and budget. I had a full-time job and was trying to fit them in. Then someone walked into our office and asked if they could leave us some flyers for yoga teacher certification at an ashram. Full immersion. I know! You just can't make that stuff up. Did the universe drop me a sign on how to complete my

4

training? I checked it out. They had meditation classes, Kirtan events, and a dive into something I felt was the part of what my soul was looking for when I originally took my journey toward Yoga.

The next year of study was tough. It required much discipline and study. I began to look forward to meditation class and sang along with much joy to mantras. I was fully immersed and gained a deeper appreciation for yoga. I realized the inner journey and work toward a higher level should not take a backseat. Yes, we move and twist and turn upside down, but for what purpose? What is your intention? I began to see how the first bit of training allowed me to get better at the techniques I had already learned. Learning the proper placement of the poses is essential when teaching and assisting students, but this year-long journey was me saying yoga is a lifestyle, and each time I place myself on the mat I am seeking a moment of reconnecting to myself.

The poses will serve as clue to which part of my body or system needs work that day. For instance, if my shoulders are tight, what weight am I carrying? Have I been sitting too long at my desk? I can now check in on how my day is going or offer myself some self-care by taking more breaks or a short walk outside. What if my lower back is hurting or tight? Again, have I been sitting too long or improperly? Lower back can also be seen as a lack of support. Is help needed with the projects I am working on? Or do I need personal support? I began to tune in to the messages my body was sending.

I also want to mention that many of my teachers were women. I am not excluding men, but it was the key for me. I think, and again this is my offering, it is because Yoga is a body/feeling type of movement. Most women lean towards feeling in the body experience when moving through life. Most men or busy entrepreneurs will find the language of Yoga interesting: "Sit quiet and go to a happy space in your mind." If you are on the go often, sitting feels weird or is a big stretch. So if you are seeking to balance out that yang energy or just want to feel yourself, try yoga. You are marrying up those two energy parts of your soul... The Yin and the Yang. Yoga, a Sanskrit word for union.

During my first steps with teaching, I was also undergoing a transformational class, learning about awareness and discovering my purpose in this lifetime.

Let's step back and talk a little bit more about myself. As a child, I struggled a lot with my identity. I was the first grandchild and got spoiled a bunch. I had lots of aunts and uncles around. Life was good and of course the universe had to give me a little challenge. Perhaps again directing my soul on her journey. Being a little black girl is hard enough at times, then add in having a birthmark that is prominent and that the universe had decided to put right on your face. Well, that makes for crazy moments on the playground. I endured the usual name-calling whenever people were upset with me or needed to gain status with others. I was easy game. I got asked a lot by grown-ups, "oh baby who hit you?" Or, "oh my goodness what happened?" Only to have to say time and time again, "Nothing... It is my birthmark." It would grow into me discovering makeup and ways to make it disappear, never really being without it except around family or people I trusted. It was a pivotal piece of my identity that the day it shifted, I was too caught off-guard.

So let me tell you about this day: I had landed a job at a very nice fitness club and had been teaching in the main studio for some time. I taught several classes each week. I had come back from a weekend working on self-awareness and had an early a.m. class. My class was full with the usual students. We had a nice

Yin restorative session in a space with a mirror. Some studios like the mirror so the students can see their form during class. Other studios do not because they feel the mirrors draw you out of your body the mind engages and you also start to watch other students. This studio had mirrors on the walls on two sides. When teaching, I first show the pose, but I like to walk around so I can assist if needed and also get a feel of the room as class progresses. Once class was complete one of my students made her way up to thank me and said, "I think this is the first time I've seen you without your makeup. I never noticed your birthmark before." I don't remember my response because I was in shock. I had left my house without performing the one routine that had become a part of my very existence every day for about 20 years. What the hell!! As the room finally emptied I turned toward the mirror and the tears fell, because there she was: raw and uncut. My soul had found a way to let it go without me knowing. I called my friend BB and we talked and laughed. Well, she laughed with joy. I was still crying in disbelief. Needless to say, I did not go back. I now wear makeup when I feel I want to, and letting go of it has allowed me an internal freedom that I did not know I would feel.

I have read that birthmarks are clues from past lives. That perhaps I was a warrior in a past life and have remnants of battle scars. I am not sure that this is true but love the thought of it and that I have brought that strength into this lifetime. I also know that Yoga was solidified in my soul that day, and that moment was meant to happen in the studio with me doing something I love and that makes me feel at home in my body and soul.

Now when I look back at that moment when the words "you should be a Yoga Teacher" were spoken, I realize it was indeed a moment of grace. My soul knew the outcome and was just waiting for me to catch up.

# CHAPTER 2

# YOGA AS A LIFESTYLE

When I heard people say *live yoga as a lifestyle,* it did make me think. I could hear the mind formulating questions: Does that mean I have to do yoga every day? Does my wardrobe only consist of yoga pants and T-shirts with an *Om* symbol on them? Can I *Namaste* my stress away?

I think it finally hit me, actually when I was watching a movie on martial arts and the instructor told the student, "Everything is kung fu." The lightbulb turned on. It is living the yoga beyond the mat that makes it a lifestyle. In order to do this you must do your work on the mat, move through the Asanas and learn the teachings so that you can begin to apply them in everyday movements.

One of the first books I was asked to buy and study was the yoga sutras of Pantanjali. It is a set of guidelines/scriptures to aid in following the philosophy of yoga.

The first sutra of yoga is : *Asha Yoganusasanam.*

Which loosely translated means: without practice nothing can be achieved.

OK let's try that; let's practice!

I began to incorporate teachings into my class sessions and into my thought process. Tried to learn Sanskrit words. Breaking out in a yoga pose whenever the subject came up. Trying to show everyone what I was learning. Things begin to change. My classes had themes to them and I began to have more freedom to share little nuggets of truth with my students. My classes began to fill up and I even had students either ask to have coffee with me, ask me to text them what I read in class, or say, "your class is great," and then bring friends back to class. The energy vibration of my soul was resonating at a frequency that was attracting like individuals. Then a strange thing happened: I drifted away from yoga.

The second yoga sutra is: *Yoga cita vritta nirodhah.*

The restraining of mental modification. Loose translation: Quiet the mind.

The other sutras work to bring you back to this one and I grew to understand why it was the second and most important one. I allowed the thoughts and images of a skinny yoga bitch or a little housewife with a hobby to enter my mind, an association with this as something that was not worthy. It was a low bar to speak something that I truly loved, and it got twisted and became like a dirty word that I could not speak. If something speaks to your soul, how can someone rip it from your grasp? They can if you are not fully grounded in who you are and what you believe, or if they prey upon your weakest threat. That detour lasted about five years and is a story for another time, but you know my soul: it will not be outdone. She found a way to bring me back to yoga. I used my yoga to regain a sense of myself and yes, identify my weaknesses; but this time it was on my terms! Having a five-year experience was a deep lesson because I learned the cues my system was giving that I flat-out ignored.

I began to realize I can take what I experienced and teach. Teach my students to listen to how each day is a new step on THEIR journey. The only voice in your head that guides you MUST be your own. Recognizing the teaching of the last sutra. My loose translation of it is: we no longer look for happiness and peace outside of the self; it lies within our true nature.

So, I am beginning to find my voice again as I teach, and my living the life as a yogi has reemerged.

# CHAPTER 3

# REFLEXOLOGY? YES I HAVE HAD A FOOT MASSAGE.

I, like every woman I know, love to have my feet rubbed. If you don't, you probably get the face I get when I say to other women that I don't love chocolate. See? That reaction exactly. So when I was introduced to reflexology I was definitely curious.

It is time for another fact about me that needs to be noted: I studied nursing and received my practical nursing license in 1989. So I am very familiar with the body and pain management. To hear there was a method of initiating healing in the body with a manual touch and pressure, I was very excited to learn more. I have had many people ask me why I did not become a massage therapist, that I have a great touch. Who doesn't love a great massage? But it was not something that called to me. When I learned about reflexology, it felt more aligned.

Believe it or not, my first course or step into this world was not with the feet. I actually took a weekend class and learned to work on facial reflex points first. This class was offered by a wonderful sound therapist in Atlanta. Again, I think my soul was already planning ahead because really? Another course that was right here in my backyard? The method is designed to rejuvenate and restore (words that later would work their way into my practice). We learned to use a facial technique along with sound therapy to render a relaxed state. I practiced with fellow students. Then, once it was performed by myself, I understood why it was so relaxing. We hold a lot of tension in our face and the muscles within it. We frown, wince, cry, and many more movements that store stress energy in the face and later in the body. So having someone stimulate reflex points and add in relaxing sound therapy... Well, who wouldn't let go, relax, and eventually snore in some cases!

Yes, you can stimulate your body system from places in your face. Everyone at some point in their lives has rubbed their temples when they were stressed or had a headache. FYI: This is a Reflex Point!. Rubbing here in a nice circular motion with mild pressure calms the system. Your system may be trying to filter out something, or there's a blockage. Stimulating this area may help to encourage the release and lessen the pain. Just a small example of how connected our body is and how we instinctively know how to move energy.

I continued the facial sessions for about six months and then decided to dive in deeper. Reflexology has a whole set of systems, and with it, teachers, researchers and therapists paving the way. Reflexology points are located on the hands, feet and ears, as well. It is a wonderful modality and there are several meridian pathways over the entire body. A total information highway. The body is such a wonderful system: We are all beautifully made!

Reflexology incorporates a few theories. There is zone theory, meridian theory, eastern Yin and yang theories. Oh, and there are certain seasons of the year that can help us to tune in to

14

our systems. So much to explore! But if we start with the basics, we learn how the entire body can be mapped onto your feet. I was excited to learn that a woman named Eunice Ingham is responsible for the framework of the charts we use today. She was instrumental in the initial foundations of reflexology. Wow! We women are bosses! I dove into the history of it just as I had done with yoga. Working from the ground up. (No pun intended.)

I often look back at my path to reflexology. I did not pursue it on my own. When I was offered the chance to study reflexology, I thought of it as a special assignment and that I was so lucky to be chosen to go to learn. I can tell you that I was like a little kid seeking the approval of the ones in charge. They knew that I would learn and I would do my best at it. They were right. It was a chance to have something of my own and, coming from a nursing background, it was not much of a leap. By a leap I mean, here is a modality to examine the body and the body systems, but from a different path. I did learn it and I dove headfirst into the energy. I would create a bubble around me and my clients during our sessions. I was open to recommendations for the set-up of my room. I could and still now get lost in it.

My sessions never have the same length because I allow myself to listen for what is needed. Time is irrelevant when I am strumming the meridians and tuning the body.

It is a constant study on how energy matters. Our cells, our blood, our muscles... Everything moves and creates a resonance. Creative energy makes us who we are. It is not a simple thing to sit at someone's feet and go into a place of surrender, asking that you be able to hear what is needed; asking that they be open to receive. You must be fully grounded. If you are not, you could project your energy onto the client and then neither of you are in a space of healing.

15

We speak words and make motions but there is also so much nonverbal communication happening in each and every moment. Our body systems are also speaking to us. Reflexology is a way to check in and see where that energy may be landing. Is it stuck in the body and creating discomfort? Perhaps with awareness and intention it can be met and released.

# CHAPTER 4

# I CLAIM THE RIGHT TO BE HERE

Deciding to go toward a holistic, more alternative modality like reflexology is a bold one. Embracing the theory that works the energy in your body naturally can feel awkward. Many of my clients come toward it first to relax. "Oh Evie I love a good foot rub! Yes I need to come see you." Then, once they are in the space, they began to understand that I am extending an invitation to explore. A chance to really explore the body and the messages it can be sending.

If they do indeed embrace this then we can take the next step, where I help them understand that consistency with your health and well-being is the way to be equipped for a long journey of life. We would not go to the gym once or take one fitness class and think, "Well that's done, I'm in good shape now, right?" We must start at the ground-up, and slowly increase our routine We must walk a mile before we decide to run a 3K.

Reflexology, like Yoga, has deep roots. There are Egyptian pictographs showing people touching hands and feet that are 5000 years old. Wow! Can you imagine it going back that far?

That is thousands of years!It has progressed and made its way to the western world. It probably falls more into a holistic, natural modality because it is outside the norm. The practitioner is facilitating, helping you and your body to release a healing response. I repeat: helping you and your body to release a healing response.

We have over 7,200 nerve endings in our feet. Also, 12 of the meridian pathways begin here. It is like an information highway. If we take a step back we can see we have always been connected to the earth and our environment through our feet. We take our first steps barefooted and began to explore the world around us. Our little toes lightly touch surfaces and we experience cold, hot, prickly, and smooth. We may start on a tiptoes at first then gradually the whole foot is upon the ground. There is a movement! When you began to place your feet firmly on the ground. And you continue to do so throughout your life. You are laying down your footprint. You are establishing your right to be here, your right to be alive! So internally you should claim your body and how it moves in this lifetime.

Listen in for all the messages your system gives you: I am hungry, Time to eat; I am bored, Let's get up and move the body; I am tired, Time to rest. If we live our daily life in real time with our system's own natural cues, we could find that we are much more in the flow of things. We can connect our thoughts and make strides in the projects we are creating. Wow! My system doesn't feel inflamed because I could hear it was time to detox. Thank goodness for the juice fast!

Along with receiving information, the body and the feet also store past experiences. Yes, some data that is uploaded gets stored. This data can affect the framework of the feet if it does not get processed out, or if we do not even have awareness that it is there. Oh!! Now we can really go down the rabbit hole, Alice. For instance, I have learned that each toe has its own story to tell about you. If you are a great communicator your second toe will be nice and round. If it is longer than your big toe, you are very talkative!

On the opposite side of this, toes that try to hide or bend over: you often do want to speak, but in the past or lately just don't get a chance. Did you check out your toes? I know you did. How close did I get?

It is your body. The one you got for this lifetime. Explore all of its ends and outs. Claim your right to be here and take care of your body!

# CHAPTER 5

# REFLEXOLOGY AND HER SISTER YOGA

It probably is not a coincidence that I became a yoga teacher and then sought out the certification of reflexology. I love the belief that we have chosen our time to come into the world and that our soul is always making its way toward our purpose.

Perhaps I needed to learn or even needed to release some of my own personal stressors or demons in order to have the space to sit and hold for someone else. When we are undergoing a mental challenge it can take its toll on the body just as much as a physical one. And yes, it feels crazy to ask the person to do a yoga session when they are stressed, but it moves the energy. I have had many a day that I dragged myself into a yoga class as a student, not really wanting to practice that day. Without fail, every time I left I was relaxed and in some ways more energized to tackle what was before me. I had the space to think and just pause for a second.

I already know about the body systems from nursing. I have had my share of babies trying to be born at home, machines alarming when airways are blocked, or just a simple moment when someone was able to get a nice shower or a bath for the first time in a while. I have spent time assisting, and taking the yoga was me learning a method of moving the body, the energy, and maintaining good health. Something that I can easily share with people. You can do yoga anywhere. No mat required. Now when I say I am a yoga teacher, my heart smiles.

So if Yoga was to claim a sister I think she could claim Reflexology. In yoga you are stretching muscles, exercising your lungs, stimulating your heart, and clearing the mind. In reflexology you are stimulating your energy pathways, releasing discomfort, exercising your neural pathways, and clearing your mind! See what I mean? Sisters.

As with many sisters, information is shared and crossed over. A foot pain can be located, zones are worked, and then a corresponding Pose/Asana may be added in. I tell my clients I have you for one hour; What will you do with the other 23? The teacher in me is trying to instill a life and commitment to maintain wellness. Working a system on the feet and then taking that knowledge to work the system even more with yoga, nutrition or whatever it takes for full integration. We have the power to move our discomfort and to not let it own us. Again, claiming a right to be.

I can imagine two sisters sitting together. The older one, Yoga, listening to her younger sister, Reflexology, telling about energy moving and how a pulsating touch can create a wave of information. Then the wiser Yogi will simply say, "yes, there's a pose for that," and smile.

# CHAPTER 6

## TIME TO MOVE

In numerology, the number six is associated with love and the care for the self. So it feels more than appropriate to stop here for some movement and care for the body.

Meditation is not a simple thing at first, but with practice it can move with ease. The mind's thoughts will try their best to keep you off your game, but it is only with the breath and a great rhythm that you can begin to get the mind-body connection. In this segment we will talk about a few breathing techniques, and I encourage you to try them. As I said in earlier chapters, we need to try things and be in the experience to know what the body needs.

OK, let's get started and be sure to have a timer nearby.

We inhale and exhale every day and every minute without thought. Our subconscious brain takes care of that, so when you take over, you move into a conscious driver seat. So do it!

## BREATHING PRACTICE 1:

Set your timer for 2 minutes. Close your eyes. Start to focus on inhaling deeply and follow with a long, flowing exhale. See if you can make the length of the inhale and exhale the same. Count as you inhale (1 – 2– 3), and as you exhale (1 – 2–3 ). If you have a thought that pops in, return to your breath count... One, two, three. After the two minutes, just breathe normally and sit for a moment with the eyes closed.

How was it? Can you tell you are just a little more present to yourself than before you started? What thoughts popped in, if any? Did they occur the whole time? Did you have a moment where there was just you and your breath?

The one important thing that one meditation teacher told me that I think really helped me to release the stress I had about how difficult meditating was, is this: You will never be able to really quiet your thoughts, but what you're trying to do is not run away with them. You are trying to keep coming back to your breathing, trying to create that small gap in between your thoughts.

So the thoughts will never stop, and the mind will always keep turning. You're just trying to slow it down so you can gain clarity and grab the things that are most needed in the moment.

## BREATHING PRACTICE 2:

Another great breathing technique is called alternate nostril breathing. I often have done this at the beginning of classes to help my students balance out their left and right brain. I let them know this technique helps to connect up the right and left hemispheres and neural pathways.

Research has been done and found that, throughout the day, we often breathe for an hour and a half out of one nostril. It could be left or right. Then we switch. The research shows that, depending on which nostril you're breathing in and out of, you can find a connection to that opposite side of your brain. Most people know and you will know now that the left side of the brain is the analytical side, and the right side of the brain is the creative side. So if you are in a moment of creating or working on a project in which creativity is required, check and see which nostril you are using. If it is not the right, do some breathing and sync up.

So let's get started:

Set the timer for 2 minutes. First, just take a couple of breaths. Then hold out your right hand palm facing upward. Fold fingers 1, 2, and 3 (index, middle, and ring) in toward your palm.

Now turn, place your thumb on your right nostril and press it shut. Take a deep breath in through the left nostril. Then take your 5th/pinky finger and press shut your left nostril as you release the thumb/ right nostril. Exhale out on your right side.

Inhale in on the right side and then the thumb's pressing shut; exhale on the left side followed by an inhale on the left side. Pinky finger pressing shut left side, and exhale on the right.

Keep going with this sequence for 2 minutes. Once the timer chimes, bring your hand down and breathe normally.

How was that? Can you feel that both sides are open? Can you feel the left and right brain connection?

Just taking a moment to breathe is a quick meditative movement. We get back in our bodies and reset. See? Just like that you did a meditation. You are on your way.

# CHAPTER 7

# I'M GONNA START

I think one thing that puzzles me (even I do it) is the statement, "I'm gonna start..." It can be finished with the word or words like:

- tomorrow
- next week, when the gym is open
- next month, after I get some other things in place
- when my schedule slows down
- after I get my money right and budget for it

All of these are things I have said at one time or another in my life when asked to do something that would clearly be good for my mind, body and soul. So why the hesitation? If we are told we have to complete a project for work or for a client for payment in two weeks, we would do what is needed to make it happen. Even stay up late hours and crunch out those creative ideas.

However, when we are asked to add in a meditation class or walk or schedule some self care, we pencil it in or say we will get back to it. We are pulled outward. We keep doing and doing, maybe thinking we can outrun ill health. Maybe if I am moving faster than the speed of sound, that winter cold can't catch me.

Well let me tell you a story. In reading this book, you know that some form of body movement is a part of my living style. I have always been active. I decided in my 40s to do a full-body detox and colonic series. I cleaned out my system and let go of foods that didn't serve my digestive tract. NO more dairy. Ugh! I was raised on milk and ice cream. But I made the jump to almond and coconut milk, and anyone in the room with me was better for it. No more flatulence! No more, "oops, sorry, my stomach is upset." I also gave up my microwave. No more processed foods.

Hearing this, you would say, okay, you got yourself on track you started. Yes, I did. But there was one more step to take: Get some labs run. I feel better, but how is my body really doing? It was a great surprise and a small slap to learn my cholesterol was high. How is that possible? I am not overweight. I have begun to eat better. Well, news flash! You can't outrun genetics. I had peeled off a top layer in my journey to better health, but a nice check-in gave me the next layer. So now I am better informed.

How does that connect with the statement "I am gonna start"? Well, if I had not started to move toward yoga or reflexology, I would not be listening or have any awareness around the ups and downs of my body, my system. If I had not detoxed my system, I may have lived with daily gas and bloating. How much damage would that have done to my internal system? High cholesterol runs in my family, and I am confronting that.

Did you hear the words? I am confronting that. I am not waiting for someday. Waiting for the day when I can lay out all the reasons why I didn't start, and seeing how insignificant they will be if I am having a health crisis. Some things are unforeseen, but I will do my best to be in charge of the things I can control. Claiming my right to be here! To live each day to the fullest.

So when someone asks you when will you start, what will your answer be? If it is not now, is that reason real or perceived?

There are days when I am prepping for yoga class that I sometimes feel tired or wish it was on a different day, but I can count on one hand the times afterward that I regretted the class. It has made me recognize that stress and discomfort was tied up in my body, my muscles and joints. The stretch of the yoga and release gives way for my soul to breathe. I am more at peace and clear.

In reflexology, I am on the giving end. Again there is energy tied up and helping to facilitate a release is its own reward. My clients can get on with the creative things in their lives and not have some layer of stress create unwellness. They gain awareness of their bodies and how they function in this world.

Okay, this chapter was a bit more serious. It was meant to be. I want to live until a very ripe old age, and I wish that for everyone. We deserve to be able to experience life to its fullest. So keep flexible, gain strength, learn to stimulate your meridians and distress.

If Reflexology and her sister Yoga where to sit down with you and chat, you would see they mean you no harm. They are delighted that you are ready to explore and that you see you are worth the quiet moments. They will gently encourage when you try to do that forward fold and stretch our your legs and back and chuckle when you say, "I could always do that!"

My hope is that I have given you a space to contemplate. Space to see there are no limits.

A space for self care to come in and have a seat.

# CHAPTER 8

# THE MAPPING OF THE FEET

It is amazing! The body is amazing. There are so many information pathways, and I fell in love with the use of reflexology. This is not a new modality. As I said in Chapter 4, it has its roots and indications all the way back to 5,000 years ago.

Just picture it: Someone after a long day of walking or hunting, reaching down to rub their feet and experiencing the relaxation and comfort it brought to the body. Then, OH MY GOODNESS! It went to the next level, when a partner or loved one took that person's foot and gave love and attention. You are there, aren't you? Your body is already connecting to that sensation, that release of stress.

Then we come forward in years, where therapists and researchers have really begun to explore the feet. They run experiments and watch the outcomes and results of their clients. Soon, we have the map of the body systems on the feet (hands, face, and ears, as well). Even though this may still bring a question mark for some, we have to recognize that the body is complex system. You eat and digest food, and the nutrients move through the body

31

and blood vessels where they are useful. This all happens without us thinking about it or making a command for our stomach to empty.

So if you are in a reflexology session and your practitioner notices something at your stomach reflex, could creating pressure, a sensation or stimulation on a stomach reflex of the foot, send a message to your stomach? Yes! It could activate a response. If we take it one step further, you now have knowledge that your stomach was speaking. Now your awareness is on this and you begin to make the mind-body connection. You now pay attention to what foods you eat and what is nourishing and good for your system. The reflexology has done its work.

What is that statement? Knowledge is power!

You have empowered yourself to take charge of your health. You have come to the table of wellness and began to develop your own by-laws. By taking a moment to get back into your body and letting go of that fight or flight response, you allow the body to give nourishment to the other systems. Your immune system will be able to function, your blood pressure may drop because there isn't a DEF CON 4 alert currently active.

In a reflexology session, I will use manual techniques. Usually, the use of the thumb and fingers. There may be some movements of relaxation, but I am working the body systems and reflexes, listening and feeling for indicators from the body on what needs attention. If we have something going on in our lives or with our health, it stores itself in the body. If the body cannot process it or move it, it will show up as inflammation, pain, or something more serious.

Often, we need some assistance to help move it. Someone else to hold the space for us as we work through what is really the root cause of the discomfort.

We listen to all kinds of news, talk shows and get advice from friends. Why not have a moment to check in and listen to what your body has to say? Ultimately, it is you connecting with you. If you were to start a project or develop something, what would you do? You would build a foundation. You would start from the ground and build upward. Well, foot reflexology is just that. We are starting at ground level.

Ok, so let's take a look at the mapping of the feet. (Add a photo at the back**) I have included my own version of this chart with an overlay on my own foot.

When I am with my clients, I share with them a mapping of the feet. I have a chart in my room. I also have a foot model that I purchased. It helps them to get visual of the places on the foot, and to understand the flow of energy within the reflexology session

As you can see, we start at the top with the toes and the brain/head. It is also the place of the sinuses. I had a great Aha! moment when an instructor said to me, "in the morning, when you make that morning trip to the bathroom and your toes touch that cold floor, what are the first things you notice?" I take a breath in because my nose begins to feel runny. Sinus reflex, ya'll! Tips of the toes.

Okay, then move down and notice your lung reflex: ball of the feet. Well ladies, the feet definitely start to talk when you wear those high heels. Not only have you taken your spine out of whack, you probably do feel like you can't breathe. Take those shoes off and, Ahh!

Now the digestive system, in the middle of the foot. The spine, along the medial edge. You are seeing how we are working the body. Working to bring the system in balance with a reflexology session. This is why I love it. Together, my client and I are on a mission to create a transformation. What happens in the body will ripple into the life and ignite the soul.

I am glad I was led to reflexology. It opens the door to discovery of the body and of the self. Yes, we may need some medical intervention for some things at some times. However, if you have a role in your health and a desire to move toward wellness, nothing can stand in your way.

So take this chart or go and explore others on the web. Take a look at your feet when you are undergoing something; watch any changes as you move through it. Get a reflexology session and get some ground-floor information or validation of what may be occurring.

One of my main questions that I often ask is: The body is speaking...are you listening?

# CHAPTER 9

## MY JOURNEY

I want to jump back a bit with my journey to reflexology. I think in the beginning I thought I would just take a course and, Bam! I am a reflexologist! It is a growing field. I talked about how I signed up for a couple of courses. I first learned a technique for facial stimulation of reflex points and I began working with clients with the techniques I had learned. Then I took an integrated course to learn the feet and a small technique for the hands. Couple this with my nursing license; I felt I would be in okay shape.

I felt good saying yes, I have a certification in reflexology, and letting people begin to book sessions with me. It wasn't until I began to get more exposure to other reflexologists and the world of reflexology that I realized something was up. My first encounter with other reflexologists who had been working for some time felt like I was under a microscope. I thought they were snobs. They gave a lot of credentials and wanted to know where I studied... and blah blah... Now my head and body are spinning. My confidence around how great this was going and what a benefit it was providing my clients began to have cracks in it. I felt like I wanted to change the name of what I was offering; perhaps I didn't measure up. However, the people who were around me were so super supportive and said things like:

"Aren't you a nurse? Then you probably know more about the body than just the feet. You have more room to assess."

"You are working within the scope of what you learn right? So you are not crossing any lines. Girl! You are great at this...keep going!"

So, I buried the worry for a while and kept working, and then decided to take more classes. Dove in deeper. One thing that applies here to the reflexology training (and for my yoga training, as well) is that it is a good idea to have multiple teachers and multiple styles. I have in both areas had teachers who were all about the rules and proper techniques. Then I had the ones who said they go by feel and create it in the moment. I think both have been a benefit.

Learning all the proper techniques gives you a foundation. A starting point. I learned the mapping of the feet and a flow to the session. Then from the teacher who talks about going by feel... I learned to try and listen through touch. Hear the unspoken words. It gives space in that moment for the body to ask for what is needed and the experience to be more personal in nature.

Through it all, I can now let go of any fear because I have the techniques and can allow myself to find my OWN flow.

So, if I am honest, I kind of withdrew a bit from the other reflexologists in my area. I was not really sure if I could fit in if I didn't go the same route. Was I ready for admission yet? But as my soul always does, it nudged me on. I took more classes and discovered there were people who did foot reading... what is that?! There was so much more to explore.

Then finally that little one in my head said, "you know, you should think about getting your full certification in reflexology. Just think what that will mean for you." So I started to think. Reflexology has been around, but it is, I believe, in in it's infancy in becoming a well-known and respected modality. Me hanging on the edge and not leaning full-in is, in a way, what frustrated me at times when I was trying to get a client to embrace it more.

Perhaps I am being a part of the obstacles, the hurdles that people in the profession are trying to get over. The more I learned and practiced with people who loved what they did and saw real results, the more I realized that I did want to be certified.

I took all the classes needed and applied to take my board exam. I do want to pause here and say that indeed was a big undertaking. I think for at least two months before, I took myself away from everything to study and immerse myself in Reflexology. I even had audio so I could listen while driving in the car. People who had taken it said, "don't worry, you can take it again." Ah no! I am going to pass and this happens now! I have hemmed and hawed too much around this already.

So the test was in the last quarter of the year and I gave myself until January to be complete. A nice birthday present. Well, did I pass? I said I would, didn't I? And I did. I then hustled to complete my sessions, some of which I had already started the year before. So, before the end of January, my board certification came!

I still can't believe it. But it is a real testament to intention, something my yogic self knows very well. Also the energy I put into it flowed back to me.

So it's official: I, too, am a SNOB! (*smile)

# CHAPTER 10

# TIME FOR SOME REFLEX POINTS

This book would not be complete without us working on some reflex points. I wanted to choose a few that are common discomforts that I hear from my clients.

So sit in a chair that gives good support and the ability for you to raise up your foot. If you are unable to do your foot yourself, read the instructions out loud to whomever you have chosen to be a part of this experience.

First, let's move and stimulate the lymph system:

Rub the top of your feet from the toes toward the ankles. You can squeeze and release or twist the foot, but mainly keep your strokes in an upward movement.

Inflammation is one of the top things that will cause upset in the body. Your system is responding to something it deems as foreign and sending troops in the form of fluid to that area. Because we are subject to gravity, we often don't feel the swelling in the body, but notice it in the feet. So directing your strokes in an upward manner helps to facilitate your lymph system and the flow of fluid up toward the kidneys and heart for elimination.

Our lymph system works with movement. It doesn't have a pump like the heart to help circulate the fluid. So help it out! Make it a daily practice to walk, move your body, and to work your feet at night before you retire for bed. Especially if you note swelling in the evening.

Next, let's look at our toes. The toes in reflexology are the area of the brain and sinuses. If your allergies are giving you a fit, try rubbing each toe with peppermint oil or eucalyptus oil. As you are doing this, bring in your yoga breath. You are trying to clear out those toxins and breathe in fresh oxygen. Help your cells to fight off the allergens. The oils will be passing through your nasal passages as well (some aromatherapy) and assisting to open the system up. Also be sure to put socks on your feet if you are cold-natured. Each time those little piggies touch the cold surface, that nose may start to run, so keep them warm.

Next, let's give some love to the bottom of the foot, starting at the ball of the foot and just working in any way that feels good from the ball of the foot to the heel. You are now working lungs, digestive system and other organ systems. When we sleep, the body is processing our day, and once we awake the next day it is ready to eliminate the things we don't need. So let's encourage it to detox by stimulating those organs and meridians.

Lastly, let's work around the ankles and the up the backs of the calves. The ankle area is for the hips and, because it is known to be the area of emotions, we want to be sure to work it so we can release any discomfort in the system in order to get a good night's sleep. Work around the ankle notch on each side. Then again, use upward strokes from the heel up the back of the calf.

Ok, I touched on a few movements. This is just enough to give you a quick reset or nightly routine and help you to begin to bring the body into balance. The body is always seeking a state of homeostasis. With reflexology and with yoga, you are learning to listen inward. Take notice of the little signs and signals the body may give. This way, you take charge of your health and well-being. Doing what I tell my clients I am trying to help them to do: put their best foot forward.

# CHAPTER 11

# THE JOURNEY CONTINUES

It has became obvious that I am indeed on a journey with my reflexology and yoga. They have paired themselves together in ways I could not have imagined.

My teaching has taken on many different forms. I started in a fitness club and then tried some private studios. I tried once in the past to start my own classes and it fizzled out. However, now with the help of COVID I have a nice online group that I teach. I also have had the gift of being asked to teach at a local senior community. I feel like the universe is giving me a chance to see how it can move and evolve even into my golden years; bringing home to me that yes!! Yoga is a lifestyle. It can stay with you and be a part of you always.

I have learned from the body experience that each class is what you bring to it. Who you bring to it. By who, I mean: what Evie shows up. When you have a theme or intention you can create a deeper level of the practice that grabs the students up as well. You all leave with a sense of connection and a reset. Yes, you can probably feel this after any good exercise workout, but I have chosen yoga. It speaks to me and my hope is that the translation to my students is crisp, clean, and brings them a space to have acceptance for who they are and where they are now in this moment.

I don't see myself not teaching. I get as much back, as well.

As far as the reflexology, each day, week, month and year it grows. My heart smiles every time a new client comes to experience reflexology. We talk of the process, and when they truly allow their system to be open and received it is wonderful to see the results. In the writing of this book I was asked to join the American Reflexology Certification Board. It was a sign from the universe for me that yes! I am going in the right direction. Yes, reflexology is a modality that can give much assistance to the health and wellness of the people who encounter it, and I get to be a part of that.

I hope this book has given you a small touch into both of these modalities and real life example exploration. I also have a YouTube channel for you to practice with me, for those who need a real hands-on demonstration. Putting the words into movements for you.

Namaste. And remember to follow your sole!

# ACKNOWLEDGMENTS

Michele L my favorite yoga teacher who now lives in Arizona. Thank you for all of your encouragement.

Meeka my early am gym partner. Girl!!

Beth Hermes, writer and author thanks for inviting me to your Novel Approach groups. It was a great foundation for helping me gather the courage to write. Shout out to Suzanne, Debi and Gary!!

BB thanks for taking my call from the gym that day.

Sharryn, Wanda, Leonie, Elizabeth & Edeline are my mastermind ladies...thanks for the encouragement!

Much love to my sister April who has always been an inspiration.

Love to Sallie, George and my brother (who shall be nameless because who do I work for the FBI? inside joke)

Thank you to my husband John for giving me the room to explore and go out on my own.

*And lastly, to my grandson Austin! Look your grandma is a author!!*

Printed in the USA
CPSIA information can be obtained
at www.ICGtesting.com
LVHW020838270124
769471LV00151B/3433